Breathe Free

Yoga for Asthma and Chronic Bronchitis

By
Dr Rajinder K Sood

MBBS, FRCS, DLO

Breathe Free
Yoga for Asthma & Chronic Bronchitis by Dr Rajinder K Sood

Printed at :

Omkar Offset Printers
#3/3, 1st Main Road, New Tharagupet,
Bangalore - 560 002
Ph: 080 2670 8186/9026
Email: omkaroffset@gmail.com
Website: www.omkaroffset.com

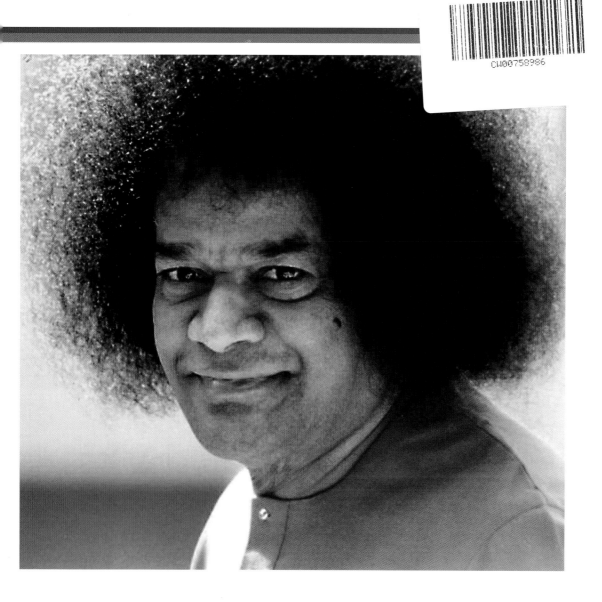

With gratitude to my divine master
Sri Sathya Sai Baba
For his benediction Inspiration and strength

Contents

Om Shanti Trust	5
Dr Sood & Dr Desai	6
Wellbeing through Yoga	7
Yoga Some Common Questions	8
Asthma - WHO Stastics	9
Respiration	10
Pathophysiology of Asthma	12
Medical Management of Asthma	16
How does yoga help	17
Yoga postures (asanas)	19
Relaxation	29
Pranayama	31
Chakras	35
Patient Responses	36
4 - Week Programme	39
Music Can Heal	43
Meditation	44
Light Meditation	45
Do's & Dont's	47
Tips on Food and Drinks	48

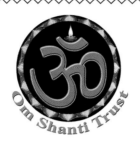

OM SHANTI TRUST

Om Shanti Trust is a registered charitable foundation. It has been set up with a view to help people suffering from common, yet serious diseases. We will explain to the public about their underlying condition, giving details of the present treatment available.

We will guide you to help yourself by following a complete yoga programme.It comprises of:

★ Simple to follow yoga postures
★ Energizing breathing exercise
★ Relaxation technique
★ Meditation

The entire initial investment in nurturing this product has been made by the trustees, Two thirds of the net proceeds are ear marked for supporting hospitals providing free medical care to the needy & schools giving value based education. We have identified some institutions in Asia, Africa, & the west.

Dr. R.K. SOOD

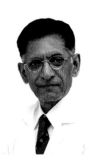

Dear friend,

As a consultant Ear Nose & Throat surgeon with British National Service in Scotland, I have seen many patients with nasal allergy and asthma.

My interest in asthma started in childhood ever since a doctor taught me to inject my mother, with adrenaline whenever she had severe attack of asthma. This action was necessary since we were living then in a remote corner of Africa.

I am a passionate practitioner of yoga and on seeing its good effects, wanted my patients to benefit from it. Making use of all information available on the subject, a detailed programme was developed for the purpose and publicity given in the local papers.

Several patients came forward for yoga sessions and they were asked to exercise at least five times a week. After several months I assessed their progress. I was very encouraged to find that every patient had some benefit.

These included:

- A general sense of well-being.
- Easier breathing.
- Fewer acute episodes.
- Some managed to reduce and even stop their medication.

Based on that programme I have produced this video and information booklet. I am convinced that patients suffering from asthma and other chronic respiratory conditions will benefit with regular practice of yoga.

Dr. Ramesh Desai (Late) MBBS., MD

He was a consultant Physician to the Mombasa, the Pandya and the Aga Khan Hospitals. He had a special interest in cardio-vascular & respiratory diseases. And established coronary care/intensive care units at the above hospitals.

Dr. Desai helped in the preparation of section on COPD (Chronic Obstructive Pulmonary Disease) and vital aspects of 'asthma.

WELLBEING THROUGH YOGA

There is a growing universal interest in yoga and the reason for this is obvious. The factory and the office worker, the housewife, the business executive, the student and the teacher have all found yoga to be useful in their daily lives.

The root cause of most of our problems, according to yoga, lies in the lack of balance between the inner and outer beings. Yoga is a way of bringing about perfect harmony in mental and physical activity.

Yoga practices have proved to be of great help in the management of conditions like asthma, hypertension, sleep disorders, diabetes, stress and many more.

Om Shanti Trust is bringing out a series of videos, which will help patients suffering from these conditions and enable them to lead a healthier life by adopting easy to follow yoga routine in their daily lives. We shall inform the public about their underlying medical condition including the medical treatment, available. We shall inform in detail how yoga can help.

We show yoga exercises which if adopted as a routine in your daily lives shall make you healthy and happy. Besides exercises, our programme suggest better life-styles as well as diets suitable for each disorder.

Hath Yoga works through the body, purifying and perfecting it and through the body upon the mind. Meditation (Raja Yoga) works through the mind, refining and perfecting it, and through the mind upon the body.

YOGA SOME COMMON QUESTIONS

Q: What does the word yoga mean?

A: Yoga is a Sanskrit word meaning 'Union' and has the same root as the English word 'yoke'. It is a union between the finite man with cosmic consciousness; some people refer to this cosmic consciousness as universal energy, some refer to it as God.

Q: Is Yoga related to any religion?

A: Yoga originated in India thousands of years ago. It is physical, mental and spiritual discipline, applicable to persons of any faith.

Q: Is there only one type of Yoga?

A: The yoga we refer to in this project is called Hatha yoga.

It consists of:
Postures (Asanas)
Breathing Exercises (Pranayama)
Relaxation
Meditation

Other Yogas are:
Karma Yoga - Yoga of action
Bhakti Yoga - Yoga of devotion
Jnana Yoga - Yoga of knowledge
Raj Yoga - Yoga of consciousness.

The purpose of all yoga is the same; to make man fit and uplift him towards higher consciousness.

Q: Besides physical & mental fitness does yoga help in diseases?

A: Over the years yoga has shown to have significant effect in conditions like asthma, cardio-vascular disease, diabetes, stress, some muscular and skeletal conditions and others.

CAUTION

☞ If you have any disease or pain consult a doctor

☞ Listen to your doctor and listen to your body

☞ Start with postures you find easy to do and move up - you may consult a yoga instructor

☞ If you have a heart condition or hypertension, avoid all strenuous postures

☞ If you have backache avoid acute forward bending postures

ASTHMA

Asthma attacks all ages, but often starts in childhood. It is a disease characterized by attacks of breathlessness and wheezing, which vary in severity and frequency. It places considerable burden on the patients, their families & the people who look after them.

The scale of the problem - World Health Organisation

1. Over 300 million people suffer world wide, the incidence is on the increase.
2. 255,000 people died of Asthma in 2005 mainly in under developed countries.
3. The incidence is between 8% to 20%.
4. In Australia one child in six under the age of 16 is affected.
5. In Germany there are estimated 4 million asthmatics.
6. In the U.S.A the incidence has almost doubled in the last ten years.
7. In India the estimated asthmatics are 20 million.
8. The incidence is increasing in most countries.

The Human & Economic burden - World Health Organisation

1. Worldwide economic cost associated with asthma is estimated to exceed HIV/AIDS combined.
2. At present Britain spends USA$1.8 billion for asthma care per year.
3. In Australia direct & indirect costs associated with asthma reach USA$480 million.
4. In the United States annual asthma costs (direct and indirect) exceed USA $ 6 billion.

N.B

This excludes some of the money people spend on over the counter medicines and treatment by alternative therapies.

Considerable time is lost from school and work.

RESPIRATION (Breathing)

Physiology

The knowledge of the normal process of respiration is of value in understanding the effects of disease and how Yoga can help.

Respiration is a complex process, which is co-ordinated by the respiratory center. The center is a network of neurons in the brainstem. It receives neural stimuli from brain and other areas in the body. It also receives chemical stimuli from the blood gases and the lungs. Most of the breathing is automatic.

During normal quiet respiration, inspiration (breathing in) is an active process and expiration (breathing out) is a passive one. The respiratory muscles of the chest bring this about. Most people don't use the diaphragm, which is an important muscle for deep breathing. There are other accessory muscles in the neck which are used in difficult breathing conditions.

Diagram of ventilation and perfusion

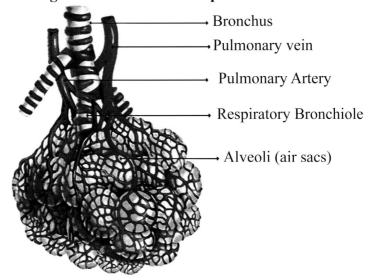

Bronchus

Pulmonary vein

Pulmonary Artery

Respiratory Bronchiole

Alveoli (air sacs)

The effects of respiration depend upon ventilation (inspired air) and perfusion (circulation of blood in the lungs). The normal adult has a pulmonary blood flow of 5 liters/minute. This carries 250 milliliters of oxygen to the tissues and 200 milliliters of carbon dioxide from the tissues to the lungs. The partial pressure of oxygen in blood is 80-95 millimeters of mercury. The partial pressure of carbon dioxide is 36-44 millimeters of mercury. Any changes in ventilation or perfusion will affect these values. In asthma and other cardio-respiratory conditions these values change.

Observation of these changes is important in assessing the nature and severity of the disease.

The normal ventilation is 6-liters/minute. Not all the volume of inspired air takes part in the gas exchange in the lungs. Some of each breath stays in the air passages (trachea, main bronchi and bronchioles). This accounts for anatomical dead space. Under - perfusion of certain areas results in physiological dead space. Combination of anatomical dead space and physiological dead space leads to some inefficiency in respiration.

This does not matter in normal circumstances because of the considerable reserve capacity. Yoga breathing exercises help overcome this inefficiency in health and during ill health.

A peptide respiratory link is well established. By conscious effort you can cause the peptides to diffuse rapidly throughout the cerebrospinal fluid. This can have significant effect on respiration. This can be done through various Yoga breathing exercises like:

- Slow deep breathing using diaphragm
- Rapid shallow breathing like pumping
- Breath holding, both internal and external
- And many more

Much of the body activity is autonomic, unconscious, but our conscious mind can enter the network and play a very important role

---

PATHOPHYSIOLOGY

Asthma is a multi factorial condition. It can occur in allergic children who may also suffer from skin conditions. Generally their condition improves in late teens. It can also affect adults at almost any age. Some people have late onset asthma. Asthma may run in families. Often allergic asthma is associated with nasal allergy and nasal polyps. The common causes are: -

ALLERGY
Pollens
(Grass, flowers and trees)
House dust mite
Foods
(mainly dairy products, eggs, fish & fruits)
Feathers
Fungal Spores
Aspirin
Some drugs
Animal Dander
(cats & dogs)

AGGRAVATING FACTORS
Pulmonary infections
Exhaust fumes
Stress
Dust
Cigarette Smoke
Exercise (generally strenuous)

OCCUPATIONAL
Minerals
Microbial (antibiotics etc)
Farming

ALLERGIC REACTION

Allergic reaction results in outpouring of active chemicals. These produce oedema (swelling) and secretions. This causes the narrowing of the bronchioles producing difficulty in breathing. The narrowing of air passages also occurs in other conditions like chronic bronchitis. Allergic asthma is episodic. In later stages when permanent changes occur in the lungs there is breathlessness even when inactive.

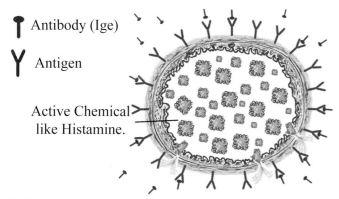

Antibody (Ige)

Antigen

Active Chemical like Histamine.

Body immune system is meant to protect us. However, in allergy, the body identifies harmless substances like pollens etc as harmful and produces an abnormal response.

The effect depends upon the site (or organ) involved. In asthma, it is the respiratory passages. The immune system depends upon the antibodies, immunoglobulins, produced by white blood cells. There are several. The most important immunoglobulin in allergy is called immunoglobulin E (IgE). This immunoglobulin (antibody) attaches itself to the surface of mast cell.

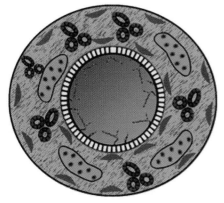

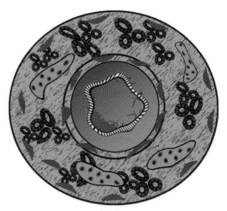

Normal Airway   Allergic Reaction

Mast cell is a large cell present in lining of respiratory passages and elementary tract. When a "harmful" substance is inhaled/ingested the immunoglobulin logs onto the antigen. Antigen is the protein present in the pollens etc. Antigen/antibody contact takes place on the surface of the mast cell. This union sets in motion a chemical reaction causing the mast cell to release strong chemicals (histamine and others). These chemicals produce inflammation, oedema & excess mucous.

Abnormal pulmonary gas exchange is an inevitable consequence of obstructive airway disease. In the initial stages the patients tend to hyperventilate. Associated stress also contributes to hyperventilation. The breathing becomes rapid and shallow. This leads to reduced oxygen (O_2) pressure in blood (hypoxemia) and also reduction in blood carbon dioxide (CO_2). In chronic conditions, these values alter resulting in reduced O_2 and increased CO_2 in the blood.

Symptoms

In the early stages there is cough on exercise or laughter. There is excess sputum production and a feeling of tightness in the chest. There are occasional brief periods of shortness of breath. Later on these periods become more frequent and prolonged. If the episode does not subside in spite of routine measures the patient is said to be in status asthmaticus. Here hospitalisation may be required. Stress, dust and smoke can aggravate symptoms.

Pulmonary function tests

FEV1 is the measure of Forced Expiratory Volume in one second. Patient is asked to take in as deep a breath as possible and then expel it as hard and as fast as possible in one second.

FVC (Forced Vital Capacity)It measures the total capacity. After taking in a full breath, the patient is asked to expel it as hard and as fast as possible till no more gas can be expelled. FEV/FVC percentage is reduced in asthma and chronic bronchitis. The normal ratio is 65-80%. In asthma and in chronic bronchitis it can be down to 40% or less.

In clinical practice Peak Expiratory Flow Rate (PEFR) can be measured by patients themselves by an instrument called Spirometer or peak flow meter. Blood gas analysis is required only in serious cases.

C O P D (Chronic Obstructive Pulmonary Disease)

COPD may be the result of repeated chest infections in a patient with poor immunity, as in allergies. It can also be caused by prolonged exposure to fumes and industrial dust. Even frequent attacks of asthma, not treated adequately, can result in chronic obstruction. Chronic obstruction may lead to emphysema. Some of these patients are breathless even at rest; others may become breathless with little exertion. They will require regular medication and breathing exercises. The carefully selected breathing exercises (Pranayama) are even more important in these cases.

STRESS AND ASTHMA

Stress is a common trigger for asthma. Stress and anxiety sometimes makes one feel short of breath and may cause asthma symptoms to become worse There are many reports suggesting that stressful life events, family problems and a behavior pattern that increases psychological conflict may influence the development or relapse of asthma and influence its clinical course. Depression is known as one of the risk factors of fatal asthmatic attack. In laboratory studies, about 20% of asthmatics were considered reactors who showed an airway change after exposure to emotional stress

Unfortunately physicians and health care workers don't address the problem adequately. Modern medical practice relies too heavily on medicines to deal with the disease. Very little emphasis is placed on the stress the disease may cause.

NOTE :

Please remember that all medicines have some side effects. Some of these effects can be serious. Doctors have to balance the advantages against side effects.

Some people rely upon homeopathic preparations. A few patients may benefit from hyposensitisation, only if a single allergen is involved. Some patients benefit from physiotherapy.

MEDICAL MANAGEMENT OF ASTHMA AND COPD

Avoid allergens and aggravating factors (smoke, exhaust fumes, dust, stress etc).

Medication: There are a large number of medicines, which can be given in tablet, liquid, injection form, or be inhaled. They fall into the following categories : -

<u>**Reliever drugs**</u> - These drugs relax the muscle of the air passages (bronchi and bronchioles) and are called bronchodilators. They are Beta2 agonist. They stimulate the receptors and relax the muscles. They are either short acting or long acting. Short acting example are solbutamol (Ventolin,Asmasal) or terbutalin (Turbohaler, Bricanyl)Long acting example is solmeterol (Seravent)

<u>**Preventer drugs**</u> - Reduce the swelling due to oedema and inflamation. They are mainly steroids. Example are Beclazone, Aerobec, Pulmicort etc.The other drugs which are an agonist receptor blocker are called Sigulair and Accolate. They are often used in children. Cromoglycate is also a preventer,. Example Intal

Adrenergic drugs

They dilate the bronchioles and can be taken by mouth or inhaled. Some can be injected during an emergency. Examples: Adrenaline, Ventolin, Seravent, and Alupent etc.

Theophylline

These relax the smooth muscles around the bronchial tubes. Example: Aminophylline

Anticholinergic drugs

Acetylcholine is a powerful substance inside the cells. Once released it has significant effect on the bronchioles. These drugs prevent this release. Example: Atrovent

Mast cell stabilizer

Mast cells are present in large numbers in the lining of the respiratory passages. They contain histamine and other active substances. Once released these substances produce inflammatory response. This drug stabilizes the cell membrane to prevent this release. Example: Intal (Sodium cromoglicate)

Steroids

They can be used as tablets, as injections or in inhalers. Injections are needed only in acute emergencies. They prevent and also treat inflammation. They can increase the effectiveness of other drugs. There are many inhalers which contains steroids.
Example: Pulmicort, Fluticasone etc

Antihistamines

Usually not very effective.

HOW DOES YOGA HELP ?

All three aspects of yoga (breathing exercises, postures and meditation) can play a role. There are several programs, which can help breathing in asthma and chronic respiratory conditions. Physiotherapy relies on gentle breathing exercises and postural drainage. Buteyko (a Russian doctor) concentrates mainly on breath holding and on nasal breathing. He believes that the main problem is low levels of CO_2.

Yoga, however, is much more than just breathing exercises. It is a programme of overall fitness, with specific emphasis on breathing. Yoga is meant to complement other forms of treatment in asthma and chronic respiratory conditions. In these conditions breathing is rapid and shallow. Mainly upper and middle parts of the lungs are used. This leads to inadequate ventilation and affects ventilation/perfusion ratio resulting in changes in blood gases.

How do Yoga breathing exercises (Pranayamas) help?

Deep breathing

It is important to learn to use the diaphragm (the muscle structure between the chest and abdomen). Slow deep breathing exercise will fill all parts of the lungs. Deep breathing overcomes the inefficiency of anatomical and Physiological dead space. Hyper ventilation is less likely in people who do this exercise.

Bhastrika (pumping) & Kapal Bhati (glowing forehead).Rapid deep inspiration and expiration help to increase the respiratory capacity and stamina. These exercises allow the body to cope with a rapid gas exchange.

Breath holding (Kumbhaka)

Both internal and external breath holding form an important part of yoga exercises. In many case of asthma, especially in early and intermediate stages low level of CO_2 occurs.

Breath holding will allow the CO_2 levels to rise. CO_2 is a powerful respiratory stimulant. Normal people can hold the breath for 40 seconds or more but many asthmatics can only hold their breath for 10 seconds or less. With practice this can be improved significantly.

External breath holding is also important. It is for a much shorter period, usually less than half the internal breath holding. One 70-year-old female patient was breathless even at rest. Her breath holding was less than 10 seconds. After 3 months of practicing breath holding, she increased it to 19 seconds and she wrote to me saying, "My breathing is easier and I can now walk up to my local shops on a windy day".

Alternate nostril breathing
It regularizes breathing. The concentration can be on timed inspiration, & expiration. This relieves tension, and clears the nasal passages of mucus. Forced alternate nostril breathing can open up the nasal passages, clear mucous and ease breathing further.

How do yoga postures (asanas) help?
All yoga postures are synchronized with inspiration, expiration or breath holding. The

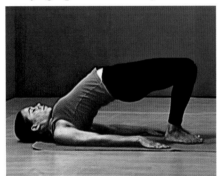

longer one can hold a posture the more stamina it gives. In later stages of asthma and chronic bronchitis there is crowding of chest ribs. Certain postures expand the chest and open up the crowded ribs. All postures increase flexibility. This makes the body feel lighter and gives a general sense of well being, which is so important in people suffering from chronic conditions.
Relaxation postures allow you to rest and breathe slowly and rhythmically. This relieves the tension, which could be an important contributory factor.

How does meditation help?
Focused visualization takes your mind off your breathing and concentrates on other

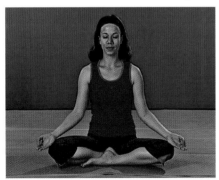

parts of the body and chakras (active centers near the spinal cord). Through deep meditation certain active chemicals are released in blood. Multiple benefits can occur. The mind becomes calm and relaxed, helping to lessen the anxiety associated with the underlying problem. Blood pressure and heart rate, which are affected by anxiety, can drop.

YOGA ASANAS (POSTURES)

In a lot of postures you are asked to stay in a position to the count of slow 5. As you progress you can extend this time. While you are in a position you are also asked to hold your breath. This will increase respiratory capacity. In most of the postures you are told to concentrate on breathing. This is very important. The asanas are to be performed slowly and rhythmically.

If you have a spinal problem, you are advised to avoid postures, which require a lot of flexion. You can safely carry out back extension postures.

If you suffer from any serious medical condition you should consult your doctor. You will still benefit from certain gentle postures, and breathing exercises.

STANDING POSTURES
Urdhva-Tadasana (Upward stretch)

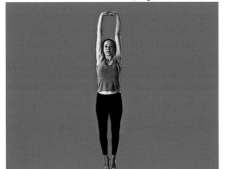

Technique.
Stand erect with feet together. Interlock fingers. While breathing in raise arms over the head, stretch up raising yourself on the toes. Hold position to the mental count of 5 while holding breath. Come down breathing out.
Repeat 2 more times .

Benefits.

Improves posture and balance. Stretches the chest and tones muscles of the upper and lower limbs.

Triyak-Tadasana (Lateral stretch)

Technique.

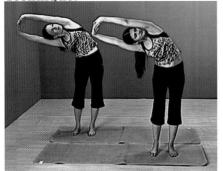

Spread your feet. Interlock fingers of both hands. While breathing in raise the arms over the head. Now while breathing out stretch to one side as far as possible. Hold the position to the mental count of 5 while holding breath. Come up while breathing in. Repeat on the other side, and repeat twice more on both sides.

Benefits.

It improves the balance and stretches the spine and side of the chest. It opens up the crowded ribs. This crowding happens in many chronic respiratory conditions. Helps to trim the waistline.

Padahasta-uttan asana (Flying bird posture)

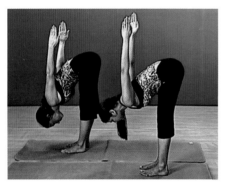

Technique.

Spread your feet shoulder width. While breathing in, raise arms above the head. Now breathing out bend forward swinging the arms backwards till the arms are vertical to the ground. Hold breath to the count to 5. Come up breathing in. Repeat twice.

Benefits.

Loosens the shoulders, upper back and spine. It will perfuse the face and scalp with blood.

Trikonasana (Triangle posture)

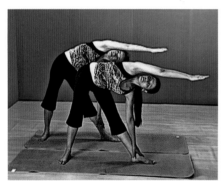

Technique.

Spread out feet wide and raise right arm above the head, pressing against the ear. While breathing out bend to the left, sliding the left arm along the leg till you reach the ankle. Stay in this position to the count of 5 while holding breath. While breathing in bring the arm overhead. While breathing out bring the arm to the side.Now raise the left arm and repeat the posture on the other side. Repeat twice.

Benefits.

Tones arms, shoulders and legs. Expands the chest and flexes the spine. Can trim the waistline.

Surya Namaskar

The word Surya refers to the Sun, and Namaskar means salutation. The sun symbolizes energy source which sustain all life on earth. Sun salutation is a dynamic group of postures. It loosens the body, stretches ligaments of many joints and tones the muscles. It also builds your stamina. It can be done at anytime (on empty stomach) but ideally it should be done in the morning. Otherwise in the evening. Try to face in the direction of sunrise or sunset (but problematic in temperate countries as the sunrise and sunset times vary widely in summer and in winter).

It is an excellent exercise and after the fourth week should be done almost daily.
It is composed of twelve postures (asanas). It should be done in a slow rhythmic sequence.

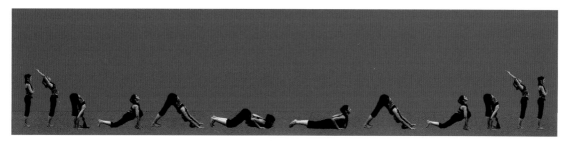

Twelve postures are:-

1. Salutation Pose (Prayer pose)
Bring both hands together in salutation (Namaskara) pose. Mentally offer salutation to the sun, the sustainer of all life.

2. While breathing in raise arms (Hasta Uttanasana) above the head and extend backwards a little.

3. Hand foot pose (padahastasana)
While breathing out bend forward at the hips, until the palms or fingers can touch the floor. While keeping the knees straight try to touch the knees with the forehead. Do not over strain.

4. Equestrian pose (Ashwa sanchalanasana)
Place palms on the floor, beside the feet. While breathing in push the right leg back. The knee may rest on the floor. Bend the left knee and extend the back and neck fully.

5. Mountain pose (Parvatasana)
Take the left foot back beside the right while breathing out raise the buttocks and lower the head. Look at the knees, both feet should be firmly on the floor.

6. Eight points salute (Ashtanga asana)
While breathing in, lower the knees, the chest and the chin on to the floor. Breathe out and hold breath for a few seconds. Buttocks, hips and abdomen should be raised.

Eight Points are:- 2 Feet, 2 Knees, 2 Palms, Chest and Chin touching the floor.

7. Cobra pose (Bhujangasana)
While breathing in lower the buttocks and hips to the floor and raise the head and chest, supported by the arms. Look up.

8. Mountain pose (Parvatasana)
While breathing out assume mountain pose as in pose 5

9. Equestrian Pose (Ashwa Sanchalanasana) Similar to pose 4
While inhaling bring left foot forwards, between the hands. At the same time lower the right knee to touch the floor. Raise the chest and extend back and neck fully.

10. Hand to feet pose (Padhastasana)
This is repeat of pose 3

11 While inhaling raise both arms over your head and extend back (Hasta Uttanasana)
It is repeat of pose 2

12. Salutation (Prayer pose - Namaskara Asana)
Finally while exhaling, come back to pose 1, where you started. This completes one round.

Repeat with other leg. You should do 2 rounds to start with. Later on you may do several rounds to increase flexibility and build stamina.

Benefits.
It is salutation to the sun which sustains us.
It is a combination of many postures.
It loosens & stretches many joints & ligaments.
It tones many muscles.
It massages some internal organs.
It gives some strength.

SITTING POSTURES

Vajrasana (Thunderbolt posture)
Technique.

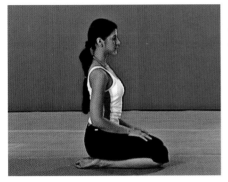

Sit with legs stretched out in front of you. Now fold a leg & place the foot under your bottom, and do the same with the other leg.

Sitting on your knees rest your bottom either on the ground between the feet or sit with bottom resting on the feet with heels turned out. Sit with the back straight, hands resting on the knees. Close your eyes and take moderately deep breaths using your diaphragm. Sit in this posture for about a minute (14-16 breaths). Concentrate on breathing. You may like to sit in this posture for a longer period. You can hold thumb and index finger as shown in the video. This is called Jnan (pronounced as gyan) mudra. The thumb represents the Universal Spirit (God for some) and the index finger represents the individual.

Benefits.
It's an excellent posture to stretch the knee and ankle ligaments. Relieves tiredness of legs as it squeezes stale blood especially in people suffering from varicose veins. Relieves fatigue after a long days work. It's also a posture in which some may like to meditate.

Yoga mudra in Vajrasana (yog mudra in thunderbolt posture)
Technique

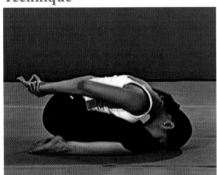

Sit in Vajrasana and hold the hands at the back in mudra pose. Bend forward at the hips to touch the floor with the forehead. Stay in this posture for count of 5.

Benefits
Stretches the lumbo-sacral ligaments. Tones the nerve plexus in the back. Massages the abdominal organs. Plus it has all the benefits of Vajrasana.

Yoga mudra in Ardha-padmasana (yog mudra in half lotus posture)
In Ardha-Padmasana (half lotus) you place one foot against the opposite thigh and leave the other foot on the floor.

Technique

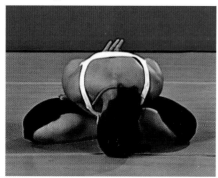

Sit in Ardha-padmasana (half lotus) with the right foot on your left thigh Hold hands at the back in Jnana (Gyan) mudra. Turn to the right. While breathing out bend forwards and touch the right knee with the forehead. Hold your breath and stay in this position to the count of 5. Come up breathing in. Repeat twice on this side. Carry out the same exercise on the other side. You will have to change to left foot on right thigh. Finally do this exercise bending forward and try to touch the forehead to the floor.

Benefits
In addition to the benefits of Padmasana it also vitalizes the abdominal organs. It stretches the spine and back of the chest. Can help people with diabetes.

Janusirasana (Head-knee posture)
Technique

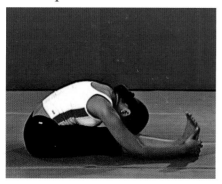

Sit on the floor and extend the left leg, bend the right leg and place the heel in the perineum. Raise both arms vertically overhead. While breathing out bend forward at the hips and touch or try to hold the foot and touch the knee with the forehead. Stay in this position for the count of 5 while holding the breath. Repeat couple of times on this side and do the same on the other side.

Benefits
Back is stretched; rush of blood to the back nourishes the nerves in this area. Hamstring muscles are loosened. Organs in the abdomen are massaged. Good for loosening abdominal fat. Holding the breath helps respiratory capacity.

Ushtrasana (Camel posture)
Technique

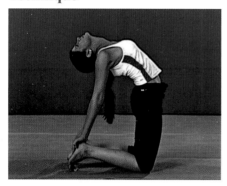

Sit in Vajrasana. Spread apart the knees. While inhaling raise yourself on your knees. While exhaling bend the body backward, supported by your thumbs in the small of the back. Keep bending till back is fully extended and take the hands off the back and place them on the soles of the feet. Extend the head fully. Stay in this posture for a mental count of 10 or 5 normal breaths. Come back to the original position in Vajrasana take rest & repeat.

Benefits

All parts of the spine (cervical, dorsal and lumbar) are extended and made flexible, can be of help in spondylitis and stiffness of the back. Chest is fully extended opening up crowded ribs, helps in asthma etc.

QUOTES

The impact of yoga is never purely physical. Yoga postures combined with breathing exercises and meditation will improve the function of many systems. It leads to distribution of bio-energy.   - Anon

"Yoga postures bring calm and balance to the body" - David Frawley

"To the mind that is still the whole world surrenders" - Tao Te Ching

A great deal of emphasis in Yoga is placed on elimination of waste. One form of waste not generally realised is tension. Tension blocks the natural flow of energy in the body. This results in disease. - Swami Kryananda

LYING ON THE TUMMY

Ardh Bhujangasana (Half Cobra Posture)

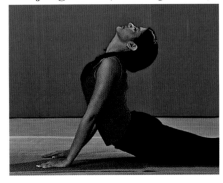

Technique

Lie flat on your tummy. Stretch legs fully. Bring hands by the side of shoulders. Inhale and raise your head & chest. Note that the elbows are flexed. Head, neck and back are extended. Hold the position to the count of 5, come down exhaling. Repeat 5 times at least.

Benefits

Gives strength to the neck and back muscles. Can relieve tiredness of the back, helps in backache due to bad posture. Increases respiratory capacity as you breathe in and hold your breath.

Bhujangasana (Cobra posture)

Technique

Lie down flat on your stomach. Stretch the legs and feet fully. Bring hands in line with the shoulders. Whilst inhaling push with the arms, lift head and chest, arching the spine. Try to extend the arms fully whilst keeping the pelvis on the floor. Hold your breath in this position for the count of 5. Whilst exhaling come down. After a few seconds repeat the posture. Perform this exercise 5 times.

Benefits

Gives strength to the neck and back muscles. Can relieve tiredness of the back, helps in backache due to bad posture. Increases respiratory capacity as it stretches and opens up the chest fully. Helps to reduce abdominal fat and play a part in weight reduction.

Shalabhasana (Locust posture)

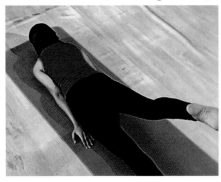

Technique

This posture has 3 stages - all, lying on the stomach.

Stage I
One leg Shalabhasana
Lie on your stomach with legs stretched, chin on the floor and arms by the side. Palms could be facing up or down, or could be placed under the thighs. After taking a deep breath raise one leg. Keep the knee straight. Hold it to a count of three or longer, and bring it down. Repeat once on this side twice with other leg.

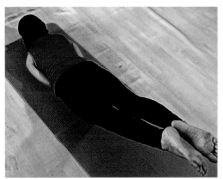

Stage II
Both legs Shalabhasana
Repeat the same exercise this time with both legs raised, chin remains on the floor.

Stage III

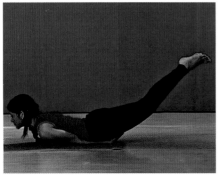

Shalabhasana with legs, chin and chest raised. After taking a deep breath raise both legs, chin and chest. Keep the knees straight and feet extended. Repeat twice.

Rest after every exercise for up to 5 normal breaths as it is quite an energetic posture

Benefits

Very energetic posture. It is good exercise as it improves the respiratory capacity, opens up the crowded ribs. It strengthens muscles of the back and the buttocks (gluteal muscles). Can help people suffering from back problems. Tones the abdominal muscles.

LYING ON THE BACK

Setubandhasana (Bridge Posture)
Technique

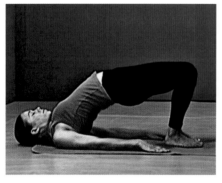

Lie on your back with legs stretched. Keep the arms by the side, palms facing down. Bend your knees and bring the feet as close to the buttock as possible. While inhaling raise your pelvis and chest as high as possible, supported on the feet & shoulders. Hold the position, and take 3 - 5 deep breaths. Come down slowly, while breathing out. Repeat the posture twice more. Instead of leaving the palms on the floor, you may hold your ankles.

Benefits
It opens the chest and deep breathing helps further. Excellent posture in Asthma and chronic pulmonary obstruction, as it improves the drainage of secretions from the chest.

Sarvangasana (Shoulder stand)
Technique.

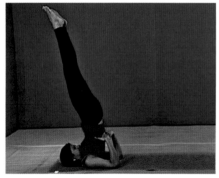

Lie flat on your back with legs extended. While breathing in push the legs up till vertical. Support the back with your hands. All the weight is on the shoulders and the chin is pressing against the chest squeezing the thyroid gland. Maintain this posture for 1 to 2 minutes (16 to 32 breaths). Repeat it twice.

Benefits
Almost all parts (Sarvanga) are benefited. It helps in drainage of sticky secretions from the chest. The circulation to the shoulders is increased. The neck is flexed stimulating cervical nerve plexus. Thyroid gland is massaged improving metabolism. Abdominal viscera are moved stimulating pancreas and adrenals. It's helpful in diabetes. Relieves fatigue and tiredness in the legs by helping venous drainage from the legs.

RELAXATION POSTURES
At the end of Asanas and Pranayamas set aside some time for the relaxation postures.

Sthilasana (Recovery posture)
Technique

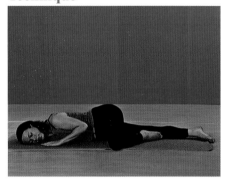

Lie flat on the tummy with the right ear on the floor and the chest also resting on the floor. Stretch out the right arm and right leg. Bend the left knee, and place the sole of the left foot on the right knee so as to cup the knee. Bend the left arm and let the palm rest on the floor at the shoulder or face level. The whole body is fully relaxed. Breathe normally concentrating on the inspiration and expiration. Chant SO-HUM in your mind.

SO while breathing in and HUM while breathing out. SO refers to the life giving energy (or God) and HUM refers to the impurities that you breathe out (hopefully the bad thoughts as well). Stay in this position for several minutes.

Benefits
This asana has many tangible and not so tangible benefits. It can relieve tension and fatigue. It will slow your heart rate and lower the blood pressure. It will still the mind and help in many ways in recovery from illness. This posture is often used in hospital medical practice in patients recovering from anesthesia, or in semi-comatose patients.

Shavasana (Corpse posture)

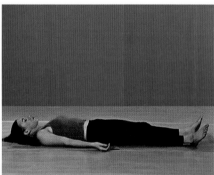

Though called corpse posture, it is anything but.
Technique
Lie flat on the back with legs and arms stretched. Some people may like to use a small pillow. All parts of the body should be fully relaxed. Keep eyes closed throughout this posture. Breathe normally for a few breaths and then start deeper breathing using diaphragm. Fill all parts of the lungs and without effort now go back to the normal breath. In your mind say SO (while breathing in) and HUM (while breathing out). Breathe in purity, breathe out impurity. Continue for 15-30 breaths (1 – 2 minutes) you may continue for a longer period. Relax every part of your body.

This is a very good asan to relax the body and the mind. At the end gently move your feet and hands. Open your eyes. Turn to to left side and get up slowly.
Sit for a few seconds before getting up.

Benefits
It is one of the best ways to rest your body and the mind at the end of exercise or a hard day's work. As it reduces tension it can have a beneficial effect on the respiratory and circulatory systems. It can have an effect on metabolism and hence help people suffering from diabetes. It can ease breathing and help to lower blood pressure. It improves concentration. It can also help people with sleep disturbances. There are many tangible and not so tangible benefits.

YOGA TIPS

➢ Choose poses that seem appropriate to your mood and energy level.

➢ Begin with gentler poses and work up to stronger ones.

➢ Breathe evenly through the nose throughout the postures.

➢ Yoga must pep up and not impart weariness and despondency.

➢ Remember the five "P's":

☞ Practice
☞ Perseverance
☞ Patience
☞ Perspiration
☞ Progression

Don't be in a hurry to go through the poses. The benefits often begin after you have maintained the pose for some time, like holding the pose for a count of 3 to 5

Yoga not only helps respiration, but lets you remain fit and flexible into old age.

PRANAYAMA (BREATHING EXERCISES)

The word prana (breath) actually means life force. Hence it implies that it is more than just the physical act of breathing. The process by which Pran is controlled is called Pranayama.

By Pranayama (breathing exercise) we regulate the vital airs in the body. This results in improved functions of different parts of our bodies. The normal act of breathing is a fairly passive process and requires only a fraction of our breathing capacity.

Various Pranayamas use our full capacity, in fact increase it. In addition the circulatory system is stimulated. Most of the time we hardly use the diaphragm in the process of breathing. In various Pranayamas we use all respiratory muscle (primary & secondary). Four stages are identified as follows: -

1. Inspiration
2. Internal pause
3. Expiration
4. External pause

Most of us use mainly chest muscles for breathing. This is adequate but relatively shallow, which becomes even shallower under stressful situations. Yoga trains us to use diaphragm fully and other muscles for deeper breathing.

Postures for Pranayamas
1. Sitting in chair
2. Padmasan (Lotus position)
3. Vajrasan (Sitting with folded knees and resting on ankles)
4. Standing

Choose the posture most suitable to you.
There are many different breathing exercises, but the common ones are listed below

Abdominal breathing
This uses mainly diaphragm for breathing. Take a moderately deep breath, making sure the abdomen swells up, with hardly any chest movement. Repeat several cycles till you

get used to it. Place your hand on your tummy & make sure it rises on inspiration & falls on expiration

Most of the time, we have shallow breathing. This becomes shallower under stress and, in respiratory conditions. The diaphragm becomes tight. This exercise loosens it and results in deeper and more relaxed breathing

Bhastrika (pumping)

In this exercise, both inhalation and exhalation are carried out forcefully. You use diaphragm & other chest muscles. There is no pause. People who have hernia should inhale into the chest only and avoid deep abdominal breathing.

Take quick, deep breaths through the nose, using both the diaphragm & chest. Breathe out forcefully. Do in cycles of 5 breaths and take a short break of up to 3 normal breaths. In the beginning, a short break is necessary. This is to avoid light headedness. With practice you will be able to lengthen the cycles. Do at least 5 cycles to start with. In this exercise the body gets used to rapid exchange of gases in the lungs. This is an excellent exercise to build stamina. If done regularly and over a period it can help in weight reduction.

Kapal Bhati (glowing forehead)

In this exercise expiration is the active component where as inspiration is passive. The breath is expelled with quick and short movements of the tummy muscles. Some people may experience difficulty in the beginning. They can learn to do it in two stages.

Stage 1

Take a deep breath in using your diaphragm fully. Expel this breath with 5 quick contractions of the abdominal muscles. Do several cycles. Once you are familiar with this technique move on to stage 2.

Stage 2

Take a normal breath in, using your diaphragm. Expel it with quick contraction of the tummy muscles. Do at a speed of one breath per second. Do a cycle of 30 breaths to start with, and repeat. Continue for 2 to 5 minutes or longer to the maximum of 10 minutes. It helps to expel certain toxins. It is a good exercise for the heart, blood pressure and respiratory conditions. It can reduce excess abdominal fat. It is one of the best exercises and should be done almost daily. It will bring a glow to your face, hence the name, glowing forehead.

Complete Yoga breath

In this exercise use all the respiratory muscles fully, including the secondary muscles.
Think of lungs having 3 parts.
Visualize the lower part being filled first,
The middle next and finally upper part.

Inhale to the point of feeling full and exhale to the point of feeling empty. Start breathing in slowly through both nostrils, observing all stages (abdominal, lower chest and upper chest). Towards the end of inhalation do a shoulder lift. Hold breath briefly. Slowly exhale to the point that all air is expelled. Again hold the breath briefly. This completes one cycle. Do 5 cycles. This exercise richly oxygenates the blood on inhalation and empties the lungs of waste gases fully on expiration.

Anulom -Vilom (forced alternate nostril breathing)

Block the right nostril and breathe in through the left nostril. Now block the left nostril and breathe out through the right nostril. This completes one round. Now breathe in through the right nostril and breathe out through left nostril. This has to be done with moderate degree of force. Normally 12-15 breaths will take one minute. Continue for 2 minutes to start with and go up to 5 minutes gradually.
It is very good exercise to clear the nasal passages, and make nasal breathing easier. Over the course of time, with regular practice, reaction to allergic substances may diminish.

Kumbhak (Breath holding)

Breath holding is an important part of Pranayama. When you breathe in and hold your breath it is called internal breath holding (Antrik Kumbhak) and when you breathe out and hold your breath it is external breath holding (Bahi Kumbaka).

Many patients suffering form respiratory conditions and stress tend to have shallow and rapid breathing. There is a fear that any holding of breath will be detrimental. On the contrary these people can benefit enormously from this simple exercise.

Technique.

Take a deep breath and hold. Note down the number of seconds you can hold the breath. This will be your baseline reading. From then on, gradually try to increase the time you can hold your breath.

After some rest, practice external breath holding. Again time it and try to increase the time you can hold it for.

Every patient who attended my clinic achieved a much improved breath holding. One patient increased internal breath holding time from 25 seconds to 90 seconds (read testimony). I don't suggest that every patient should attempt to go that far. This exercise gives a tremendous confidence to people suffering from conditions like asthma and chronic bronchitis. It improves their respiratory function.

Breath holding chin lock & shoulder exercise

Take a moderately deep breath and hold your breath. Lock the chin on the chest. Move shoulders up and down rapidly without bending the elbows. Hold the breath for as long as you comfortably can. Repeat this exercise 5 times. Try to increase the time of breath holding. It is a very good exercise to build the respiratory capacity. It gives confidence to patients suffering respiratory disability and stress.

PRANAYAMA TIPS

➤ Never strain your breathing in pranayama.

➤ Breathe deeply and slowly, except in some exercises.

➤ Progress slowly and carefully.

➤ If you feel dizzy or light-headed, return to normal breathing.

➤ Pranayama should be performed almost daily.

QUOTES

If you can't breathe nothing else matters. - Ginger Kohlman (Nurse, University of California)

The benefits of Yoga breathing exercises are often underestimated.

Certain breathing exercises if continued for several minutes (10 or more) can burn a lot of calories. Can help in weight reduction.

CHAKRAS

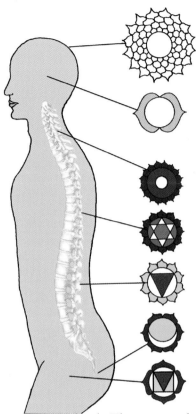

Sahasrara Chakra (Crown Chakra)

Ajna Chakra (Third eye Chakra)

Vishnuddhi Chakra (Throat Chakra)

Anhata Chakra(Heart Chakra)

Manipura Chakra(Solar pluxus Chakra)

Swadhisthana Chakra (Sacral Chakra)

Mooladhara Chakra (Root Chakra)

Chakra means a wheel. They are subtle psychic areas of energy distributed from the brain to the bottom of the spine. Yoga master believe that these centers control the distribution of Prana (life force).

There are seven major chakras. They are located around the central energy channel called Sushmna nadi (chanel). The chakras are interconnected by energy network called nadis.

Focusing on chakras while performing yoga exercises will activate the chakras and encourage the flow of energy through them. It is believed by yoga masters, that disease occurs when there is a block in the free flow of energy in these chakras.

The most important chakra for the heart and lungs is called Anhata chakra. Cardiac nerve plexus and the vagus (10th cranial nerve) are closely associated with this chakra. Breathing exercises will activate this chakra.

PATIENT RESPONCES

Report on breathing exercises for asthmatics

Early in 2001 I attended a course taken by Dr Sood aimed at teaching the participants exercises which if undertaken daily would improve their breathing ability and so hopefully lessen the severity and number of attacks.

I have kept on doing these exercises daily before breakfast and have noticed the following improvements:

1. My peak flow measurement has improved from between 180-200 to 200-230 during periods when I am not suffering from colds etc.

2. Apart from one occasion late in 2002 when I caught a really severe throat infection I managed to do my exercises

3. Doing the exercises gives me a sense of well being at my age (71) and I get a sense of relief at being able to do something myself to combat the asthma instead of relying entirely on inhalers.

4. I can now hold my breath for 90 seconds at a time instead of 25 seconds when I first started doing this exercise.

I am very grateful to Dr Sood for giving of his time in order that I and others might achieve the above.

Mrs. Rita Riddell
3 Coats Place Dundonald Scotland

Dear Dr Sood,

Before I started the Yoga for asthmatics, I had just recovered from a severe chest infection that lasted for a period of three months. I frequently suffered from bronchial spasms during the nights whilst asleep, which left with me with an element of anxiety about going to bed.

After the infection had cleared I was left with asthma, and still with the fear of taking bronchial spasms again even with medication.

At the time of getting the chest infection, I was studying in my second year for B.A. (Hon) for film and television at the University of Westminster (London) and consequently I was forced to take a year out.

I had a real inner debate as to whether I wanted to complete my studies. This was mainly due to a psychological fear of the same thing happening again.

However, having attended the Yoga for Asthmatics and worked on it for a few months prior to going back to university, I found that my general breathing was a lot stronger and physically I was more healthier than even prior to the initial chest infection. I also found that within a few weeks of the yoga I was gradually capable of taking up strenuous sporting activities again, such as football, which I had a fear of playing again.

Having regained a good physical well being after using the yoga, I eventually gained the self-confidence to go back to university, and eventually I graduated in June 2003. I would like to take this opportunity to thank you for all the help in teaching me Yoga.

Eaun Lee
22 Barra Lane Broomlands, Irvine Scotland.

Report on breathing exercises from Bruce Riddell

I took careful note of my wife, Rita's breathing exercises and noted the improvement to her well – being. Although not affected by asthma to any significant extent, nonetheless I started to copy her exercises each morning and noted that I, too, benefit from them in that I have more energy and a greater sense of fitness and general well – being.

I have continued with the exercises ever since on a daily basis. I am also 71 years of age and I have angina, which is controlled by daily medication. However I rarely have any problems with the angina.

Needless to say, I am very pleased that Rita started the course of treatment under Dr Sood, as clearly I have gained much benefit indirectly from copying the exercise

Bruce Riddell

I was diagnosed with Asthma in 1996 with severe breathing difficulties. I was given a nebuliser and inhalers to control my symptoms. I had to take a steroid inhaler twice every day even then had quiet a few bad attacks.

The real turning point came when I read in a local newspaper article about Dr Sood doing research into yoga helping asthmatics. Dr Sood taught us yogic breathing techniques which he advised us to do every morning if possible.

I have been going to yoga twice a week since our visits and I also do my breathing exercises nearly every morning. I have stopped all my inhalers, including the steroid one. I know I am still asthmatic and wouldn't like to say that I will never need an inhaler again but at the moment I am glad to be off the steroid treatment.

I like to thank Dr Sood for making such a difference to my life.   - Ran Surgenor

Dear Mr. Sood,

I am sending the result of my breathing over the last two months I feel my breathing is much easier and can walk into the winds now. My breath holding has improved from 9 seconds to 19 seconds.

Thank you for your help
Jane P Love
155 Logan Drive Troon, Scotland.

This is a small sample of patient responses. In an anonymous questioner every patient noticed some benefit through this programme.

4 WEEK PROGRAMME

Why a four week programme?
The purpose is to introduce many exercises gradually so that you may understand and become familiar with them before you move to the next set of exercises.

After four weeks you can draw up your own daily programme. It must include at least 4 breathing exercises, 8 postures (selected from different sections) Relaxation posture is in addition to the other postures.

Patents with breathing difficulties find recovery posture (sthilasana) easier than corpse posture (Sarvangasana) for relaxation.

In earlier stage you may use a pillow for the head in corpse posture.

WEEK - 1	
Warm up Exercises	3 - 5 minutes
Postures (Asanas)	Repeat all exercises 3 times or more

Standing Postures
Urdhva Tadasana (Upward Stretch)
Tiryak - Tadasana (Lateral Stretch)
Padahasta uttan asana (Flying bird)

Sitting Posture
Vajrasana (Folded knees or Thunderbolt)
Yoga Mudra in Vajrasana (Yoga Mudra in Thunderbolt)

Lying on tummy
Ardha Bhujanghasana (Half Cobra posture)

Relaxation
Sthilasana (Recovery posture)

Breathing exercises (Pranayamas)

Adham Pranayama (Abdominal breathing) up to	1 minute
Mahat Yoga Pranayama (Full yoga breath)	5 breaths
Anuloma - Viloma (Forced alternate breathing)	2 minutes

Breath holding
Antrik kumbhaka (Internal)
(Breathe in fully and hold the breath for as long as comfortable).

Bahya Kumbaka (External)
(Breathe out fully and hold the breath for as long as comfortable).
Keep extending the time you can hold your breath, Time it and note in seconds how long you can hold your breath.

WEEK - 2

Warm up Exercises   3 - 5 minutes

Postures (asanas)   Repeat all exercises 3 times or more

Standing Postures
Urdhva Tadasana (Upward Stretch)
Tiryak - Tadasana (Lateral Stretch)
Padahasta uttan asana (Flying bird)

Sitting Posture
Yoga mudra in Vajrasan (Yoga mudra in folded knee posture)
Yoga mudra in Ardha padmasana (Yog Mudra in half lotus posture)
Janusirasana (Forehead knee posture)

Lying on tummy
Bhujangasana (Full Cobra posture)

Lying on Back
Setubandhasana (Bridge pose)

Relaxation
Sthilasana (Recovery posture)

Breathing exercises (Pranayamas)
Adham Pranayama (Abdominal breathing) upto   1 minute
Mahat Yoga Pranayama (Full yoga breath)   5 breaths
Kapalbhati - Slow (Shining forehead breathing) 2 minutes

Breath holding
Antrik kumbhaka (Internal) Breathe in fully and hold the breath for as long as comfortable
Bahya Kumbaka (External) Breathe in fully and hold the breath for as long as comfortable. Keep extending the time you can hold your breath, you may like to time it and note in seconds how long you can hold your breath.

WEEK - 3	
Warm up Exercises	3 - 5 minutes
Postures (asanas)	Repeat all exercises 3 times or more

Standing Postures
Urdhva Tadasana (Upward Stretch)
Trikone asana (Triangle pose)
Padahastna uttan asana (Flying bird)

Sitting Posture
Yoga mudra in Ardha padmasana
(Yog Mudra in half lotus posture)
Janusirasana (Forehead knee posture)

Lying on tummy
Bhujangasana (Full Cobra posture)

Lying on Back
Sarvangasana (Shoulder stand)

Relaxation
Sthilasan (Recovery posture) or
Shavsana (Relaxation posture)

Breathing exercises (Pranayamas)

Bhastrika (Pumping)	5 cycles of 5 breath each and extend
Anulome - Vilome (Forced alternate breathing)	2 minutes
Kapalbhati - Slow (Shining forehead breathing)	2 minutes

Breath holding

Antrik kumbhaka (Internal) Breathe in fully and hold the breath for as long as comfortable.

Bahya Kumbaka (External) Breathe out fully and hold the breath for as long as comfortable.

Keep extending the time you can hold your breath, you may like to time it and note in seconds how long you can hold your breath.

WEEK - 4

Warm up Exercises   3 - 5 minutes

Postures (asanas)   Repeat all exercises 3 times or more

Standing Posture
Surya Namaskara (Sun Salutation)

Sitting Posture
Vajrasana (Folded knees or kneeling)
Yoga mudra in Ardha padmasana
(Half lotus posture with yog mudra)
Ushtrasana (Camel pose)

Lying on tummy Posture
Salabhasana

Lying on Back
Shoulder stand (Sarvangasana)

Relaxation
Shavasana (Relaxation Posture)

Breathing exercises (Pranayamas)
Mahat Yoga Pranayama (Full Yoga Breath)   5 times
Bhastrika (Pumping)   5 cycles of 10 breath each and
                                               extend
Anulome - Vilome (Forced alternate breathing) 2 minutes
Kapalbhati - Slow (Shining forehead breathing) 2 minutes

CONGRATULATIONS!

With this you have completed four week training programme. By now you will be familiar with all the exercises. All exercise are important. You should draw up your daily plan to include some exercises from each section. Yoga and meditation will make you whole very quickly.

You will feel more confident and relaxed.

Do not neglect your normal medication. However over the course of time you will require less medication. Keep consulting your physician.

THERAPEUTIC MUSIC

The ancients were aware of the fact that music can heal and the moderns are now putting this fact to good use such as curing and alleviating a variety of diseases, from Hypertension to Cancer. How exactly this takes place is still not fully understood, but there are excellent hypotheses.

"Non physical sound tackles the physical ills through the non-physical mind of each one of us"

3rd B.C Ayurved Acharya Vedeve Dutt reflected on this as ——
"The best doctors heal with the divine sound" fact and putting it to good use.

Five hundred year ago " The holy guru granth sahib" invoke ——
"Sarv rog ka aukhad naam"
"Sound is the medicine for all the ailments"

 18th Century Mystic Novalis states
"Every ailment is a musical problem and cure lies in musical solution" most elusive.

Sound vibrations are an eternal garment of everything from pebble to piano keys. Everything is born with a certain vibrational character and form an interdependent web woven out of multi-dimensional mental impulse threads. Problems (dis-ease) start encroaching upon our normal ease when there occurs a shift or change in our inherited vibrational character (The Pitch). With angry mood it will shoot up and with depression it will go down the ladder of chromatic scale and will disturb the normal behaviour of living melody. With the general above noted conditions the flow of music or sound vibrations transfer movement to statically pestering thoughts of disease and localized pain through feelings by steering the mind towards an optimum release, relief being given by the touch of harmonious chords of meditation.

The right type of music should be played while doing yogic asanas so that it enhances the healing process. Similarly, meditation becomes all the more effective if accompanied by suitable music. The benefits of music therapy in relieving stress and improving relaxation are widely accepted, as is its value in the well being of children and the elderly. Some studies have shown that music can affect the rhythm of breathing and heartbeat, and can alter blood pressure. Music is a great antidote to the stress of life today - whether you play a favorite CD, attend concert recitals or play an instrument – the therapeutic benefits of music can calm even the most troubled mind.

MEDITATION

After seating oneself in a comfortable & stable posture, steadying your breath, & stilling your mind purification of all the organs of the body is done.

Light is the greatest purifier for it dispels all darkness.

We start by visualising light travel through the body, purifying all the limbs and senses.

Within a few days of meditation the mind will be more controlled and you will taste the joy of concentration.

It is important to reflect upon the peace and joy you experience during meditation

After meditation, do not get up suddenly and start moving around, resuming your activities. Loosen your limbs slowly, deliberately and gradually before you enter upon your usual duties.

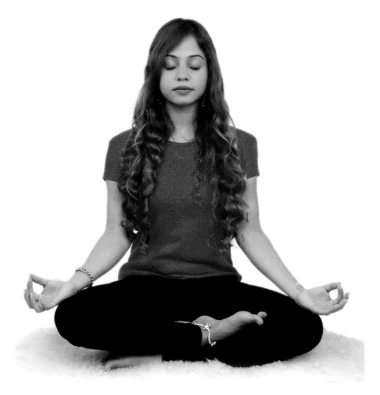

LIGHT MEDITATION

Light meditation is the most universal and the most effective form of meditation. It is the first step in spiritual discipline. At first, set aside a few minutes daily for meditation and later extend the time as you feel the bliss that you get.

Let it be in the hours before dawn. This is preferable because the body is refreshed after sleep and the dealings of daytime will not yet have impinged upon you.

Have a lamp or a candle before you with an open, steady and straight flame. Sit comfortably in front of the candle in the lotus position or any other comfortable sitting position.

Let us now begin, Look at the flame steadily for some time. And closing your eyes and try to feel the flame inside you centered between your eyebrows. Let it slide down into the lotus of your heart, illuminating the path.

When it enters the heart, imagine that the petals of the lotus open out one by one, bathing every thought, feeling and emotion in the light and so removing darkness. There is no space for darkness to hide where there is light

The light of the flame now becomes wider and brighter. Allow it to heal each and every part of you. Let it pervade your limbs.

Now those limbs can never deal in negative activities; They have become instruments of light and love.

As the light touches your arms and hands, let it allow you to serve and help others.

As the light reaches up to the tongue, falsehood vanishes from it, let it rise up to the eyes and the ears and destroy all dark desire that infests them, let your head be surcharged with light and all wicked thoughts will flee there from.

Imagine that the light in you more and more intensely. Let it shine all around you and let it spread from you in ever-widening circles, taking in your loved ones, your kith and kin, your friends and companions, your enemies and rivals, strangers, all living beings, the entire world.

Stay in that thrill of witnessing the light everywhere. If you adore God in any form, try to visualize that form in the all-pervasive light. For Light is God and God is light

- Adapted and modified from Sri Sathya Sai Baba

ROLE OF THE MIND

During our daily, busy lives, the mind is focused on external things. The brain activity recorded during this period shows beta waves. These waves are small and frequent (usually over 13 cycles per second) Yoga trains you to focus internally, especially during breathing exercises and meditation. These results in alpha waves activity of the brain. Alpha waves are larger and slower than beta waves. This way your mind can have a very powerful influence on your health and also on the underlying condition you are suffering from.

Several studies in America have shown both psychological and physiological benefits with regular practice of meditation.

If the inner self is allowed to work through a relaxed and peaceful nervous system it will fill the body with energy and strength. Swami Kryananda

DO's AND DONT's

Do's

☑ Use yoga mat

☑ Practice yoga in a ventilated room, or in the open when weather permits.

☑ Get up in the morning at a regular time allowing at least half an hour for yoga. Or you may prefer to do it in the evenings

☑ Do yoga at least 5 days a week.

☑ Keep your house free of dust, especially your bedroom.

☑ Keep weight under control as excess weight strains the respiratory and Cardiovascular systems

☑ Take medications as advised. You will be able to reduce the dosage with regular practice

Don'ts

☒ Don't smoke

☒ Don't overeat

☒ Don't over exert yourself

☒ Don't keep pets if allergic to animals

Avoid

■ Carpets and rugs as they trap dust and house dust mites.

■ Smoky dusty places.

■ Flowers in the house if you suffer from pollen allergy.

■ Rushing. Give enough time for travel.

■ Aggravating situations like arguments.

TIPS ON FOOD AND DRINK

☑ Take plenty of fresh fruits and vegetables, as they are a rich source of vitamins, minerals, antioxidants and essential oil.
Darker the fruit higher the antioxidant content.
Apples shouldn't be skinned, as their skin is rich in antioxidants.

☑ Some American studies have shown that vitamin A, C, D and calcium supplements can help. Some people's diet may be deficient in vitamins and minerals.

☑ Always read labels for any thing you may be allergic to.

☑ Nuts especially almonds are good, soak 5 - 10 of them over night and eat in the morning after removing the skin. They can lower cholesterol.

AVOID

■ Any food that you think you may be allergic to.

■ Processed food as they contain excess amount of salt and saturated fat. They also contain preservatives (sulphites) and artificial colours (especially Tertrazine). Some people are sensitive to these substances.

■ Cold fizzy drinks. They usually contain artificial colours and additives. They generally have no significant -food value.

■ Drugs that you may be allergic to. Aspirin allergy is known to play a significant role in some asthmatics.

With a regular practice of this programme your breathing will be easier and your body fitter and more flexible.